I Care for Myself

Katie Peters

GRL Consultants,
Diane Craig and Monica Marx,
Certified Literacy Specialists

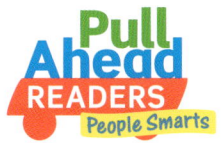

Lerner Publications ◆ Minneapolis

Note from a GRL Consultant
This Pull Ahead leveled book has been carefully designed for beginning readers. A team of guided reading literacy experts has reviewed and leveled the book to ensure readers pull ahead and experience success.

Copyright © 2023 by Lerner Publishing Group, Inc.

All rights reserved. International copyright secured. No part of this book may be reproduced, stored in a retrieval system, or transmitted in any form or by any means—electronic, mechanical, photocopying, recording, or otherwise—without the prior written permission of Lerner Publishing Group, Inc., except for the inclusion of brief quotations in an acknowledged review.

Lerner Publications
An imprint of Lerner Publishing Group, Inc.
241 First Avenue North
Minneapolis, MN 55401 USA

For reading levels and more information, look up this title at www.lernerbooks.com.

Main body text set in Memphis Pro 24/39
Typeface provided by Linotype.

Photo Acknowledgments
The images in this book are used with the permission of: © FatCamera/Getty Images, pp. 10–11; © FG Trade/Getty Images, pp. 12–13, 16 (right); © JackF/Getty Images, pp. 8–9; © kornnphoto/Shutterstock Images, p. 3; © PeopleImages/Getty Images, pp. 14–15, 16 (left); © Raul_Mellado/Getty Images, pp. 4–5, 16 (center); © StockPlanets/Getty Images, pp. 6–7.

Front cover: © TinnaPong/Shutterstock Images.

Library of Congress Cataloging-in-Publication Data

Names: Peters, Katie, author.
Title: I care for myself / Katie Peters.
Description: Minneapolis, MN : Lerner Publications, [2023] | Series: I care (Pull Ahead Readers People Smarts—nonfiction) | Includes index. | Audience: Ages 4–7 | Audience: Grades K–1 | Summary: "Making time to play, bathe, or dance is good for your health. Early readers can explore ways to care for themselves in this easily accessible text. Pairs with the fiction book, Cara Takes Time"— Provided by publisher.
Identifiers: LCCN 2021044341 (print) | LCCN 2021044342 (ebook) | ISBN 9781728457680 (library binding) | ISBN 9781728461540 (ebook)
Subjects: LCSH: Self-care, Health—Juvenile literature. | Well-being—Juvenile literature. | Caring—Juvenile literature.
Classification: LCC RA777 .P484 2023 (print) | LCC RA777 (ebook) | DDC 613—dc23

LC record available at https://lccn.loc.gov/2021044341
LC ebook record available at https://lccn.loc.gov/2021044342

Manufactured in the United States of America
1 – CG – 7/15/22

Table of Contents

I Care for Myself.......4

Did You See It?........16

Index..................16

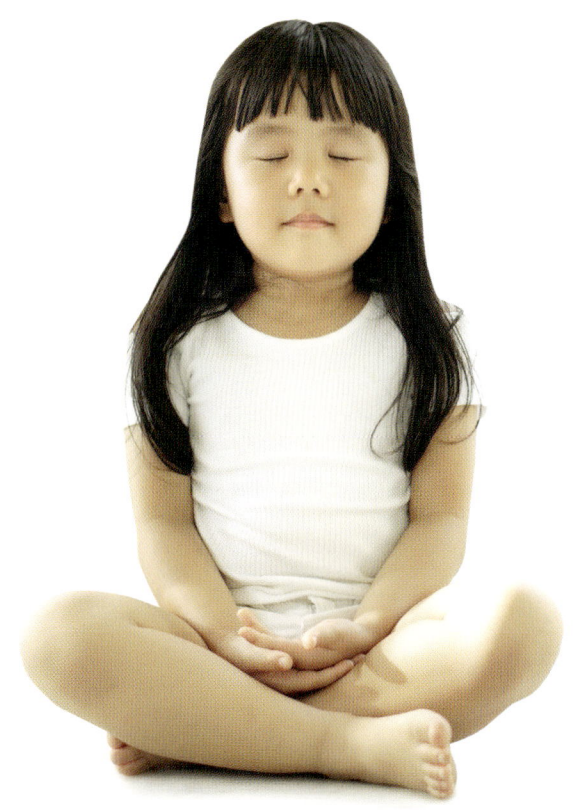

I Care for Myself

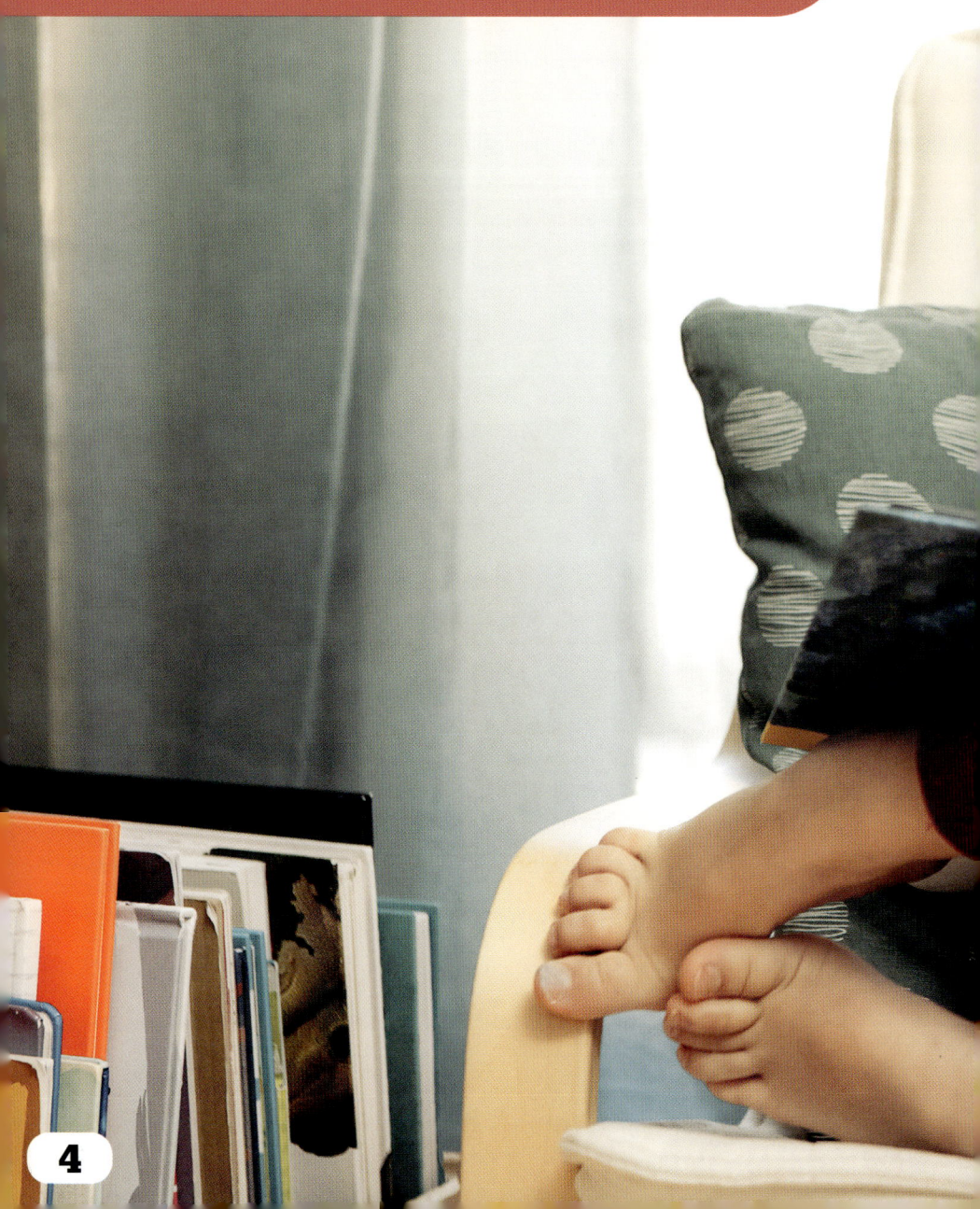

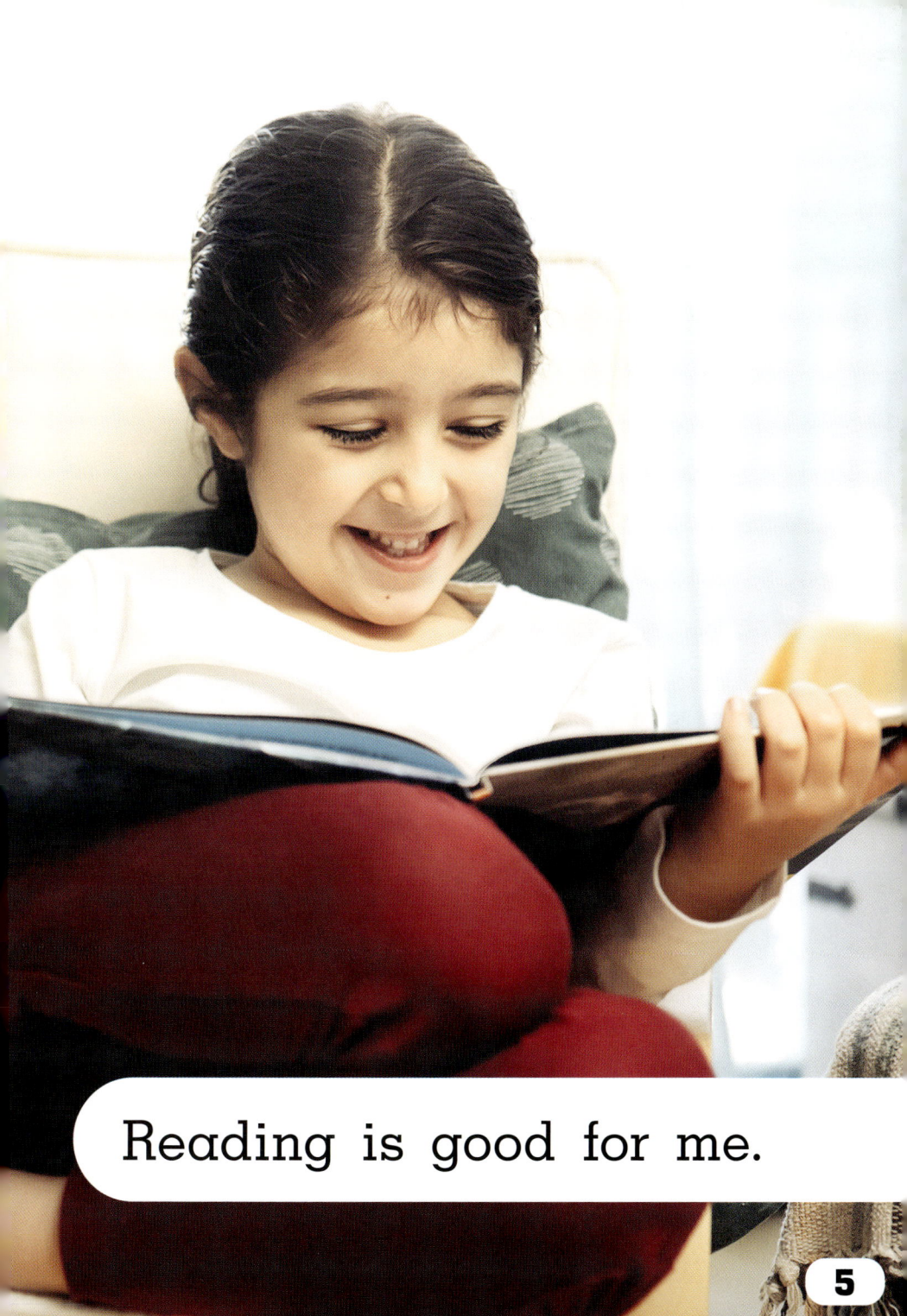

Reading is good for me.

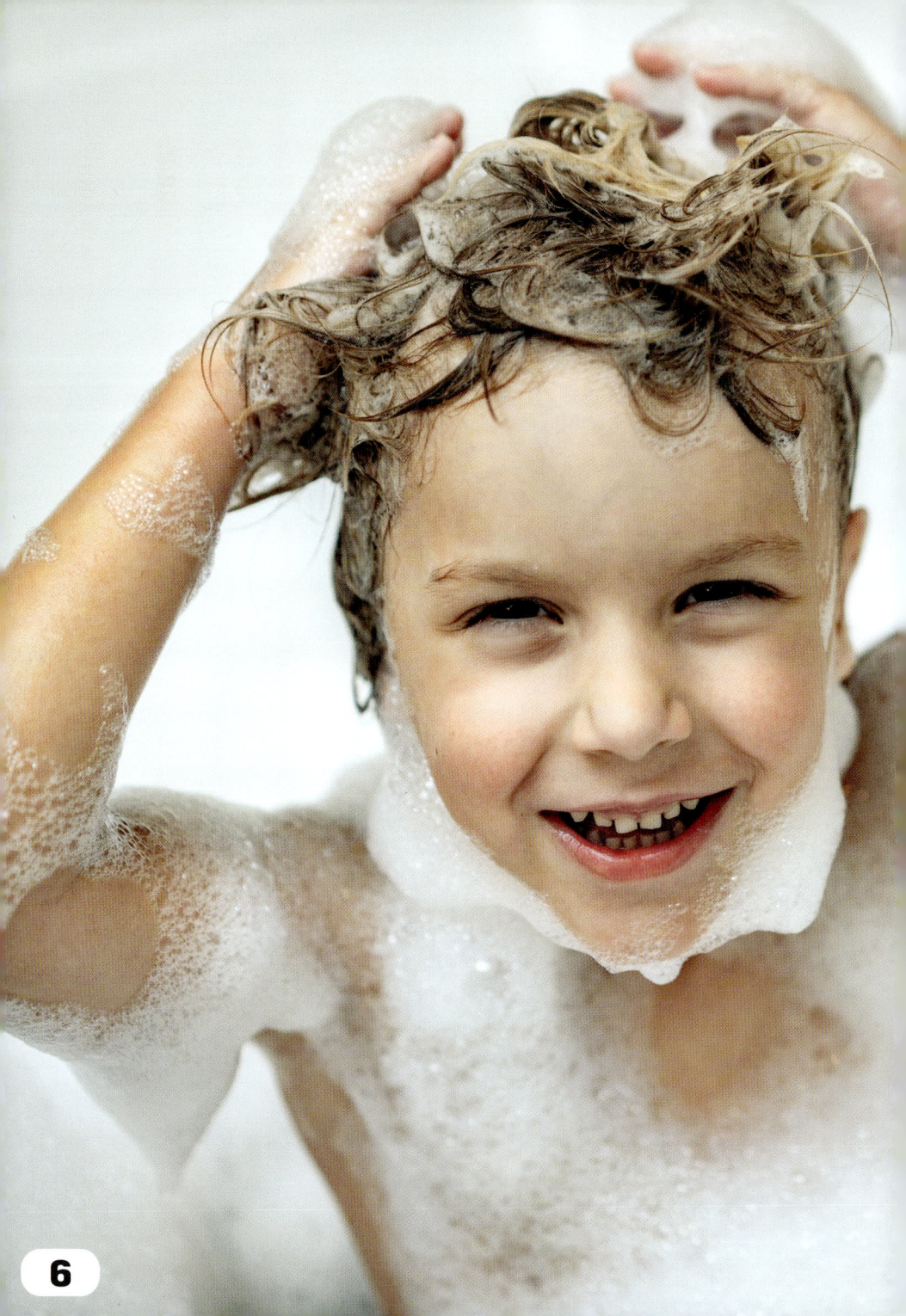

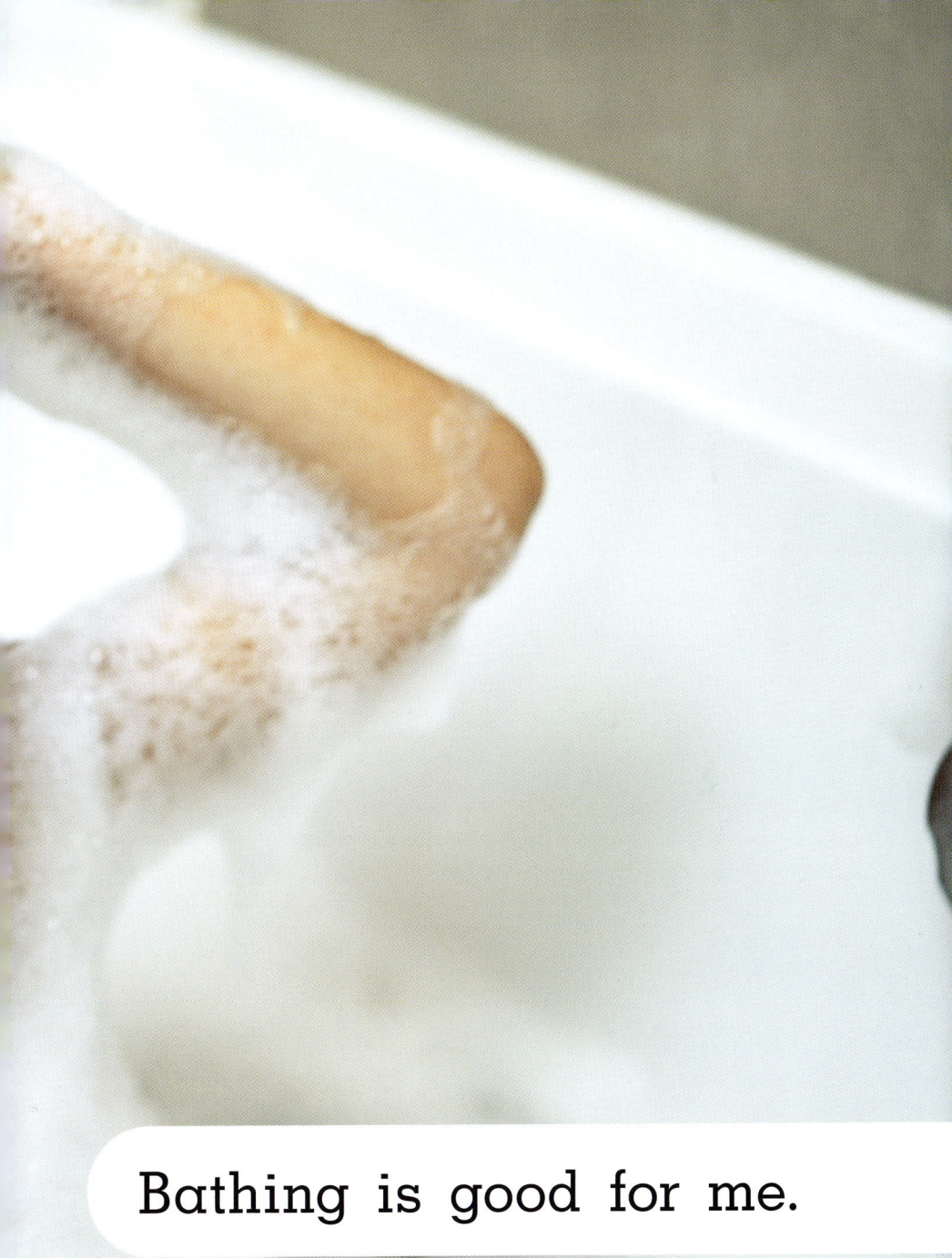

Bathing is good for me.

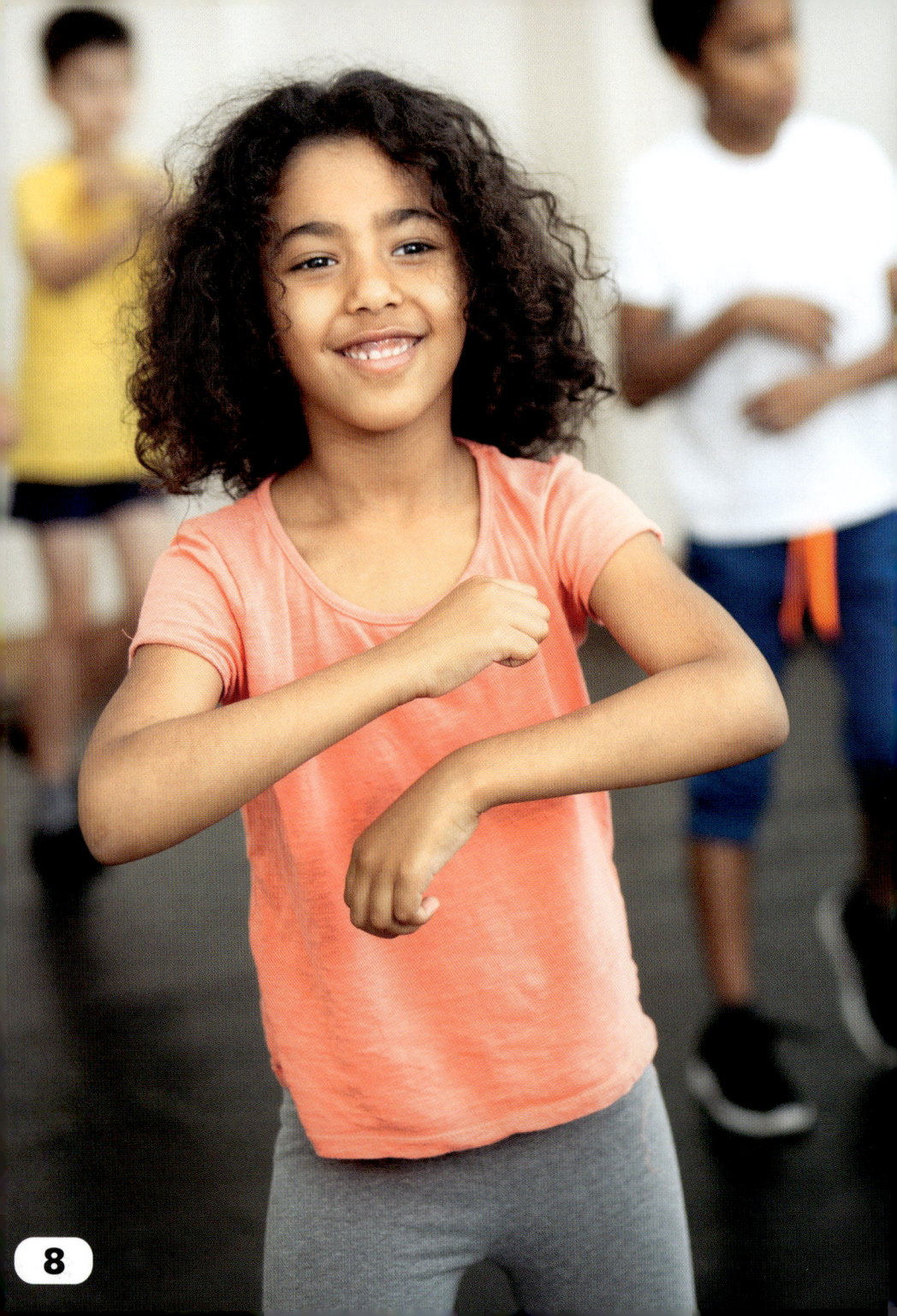

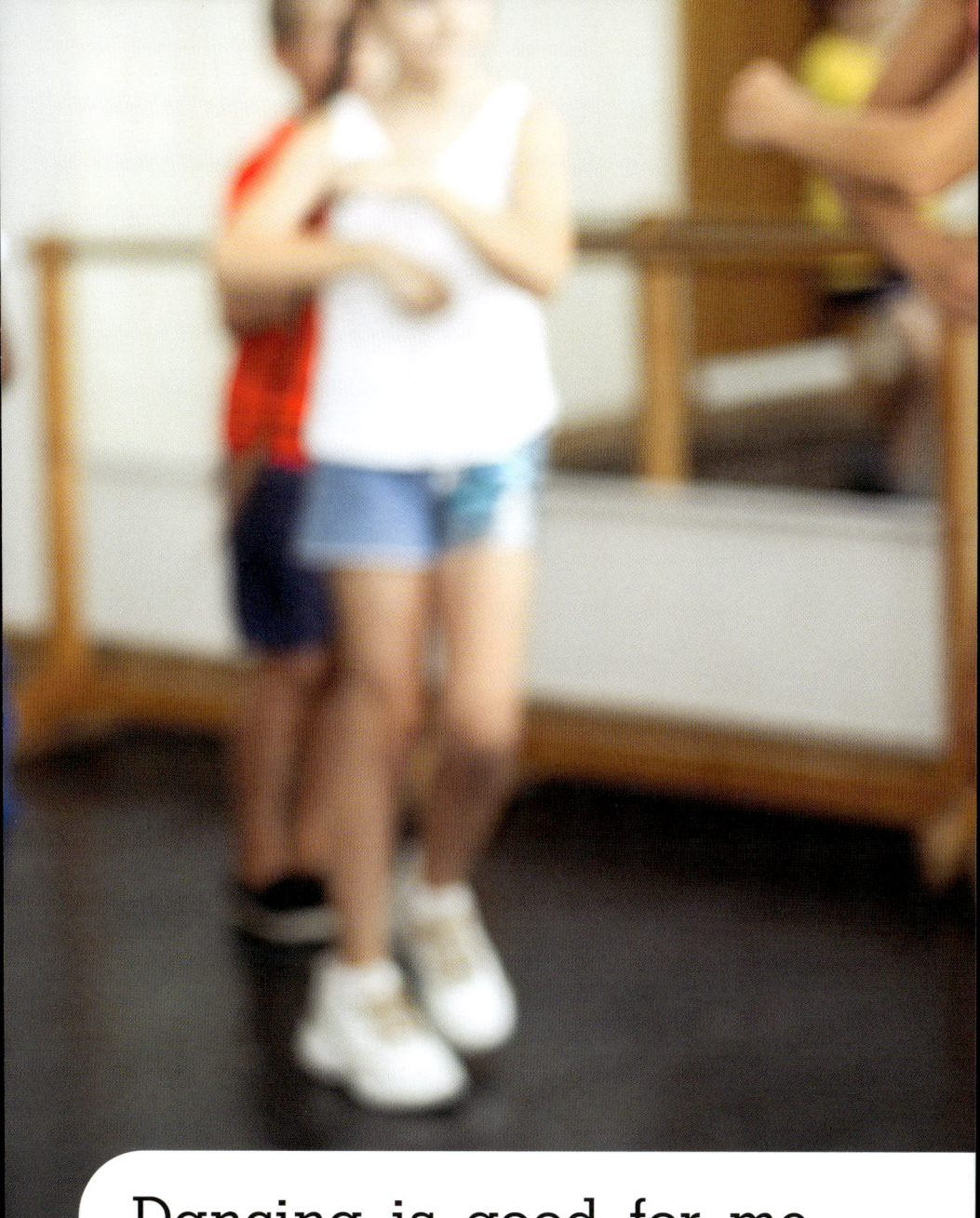

Dancing is good for me.

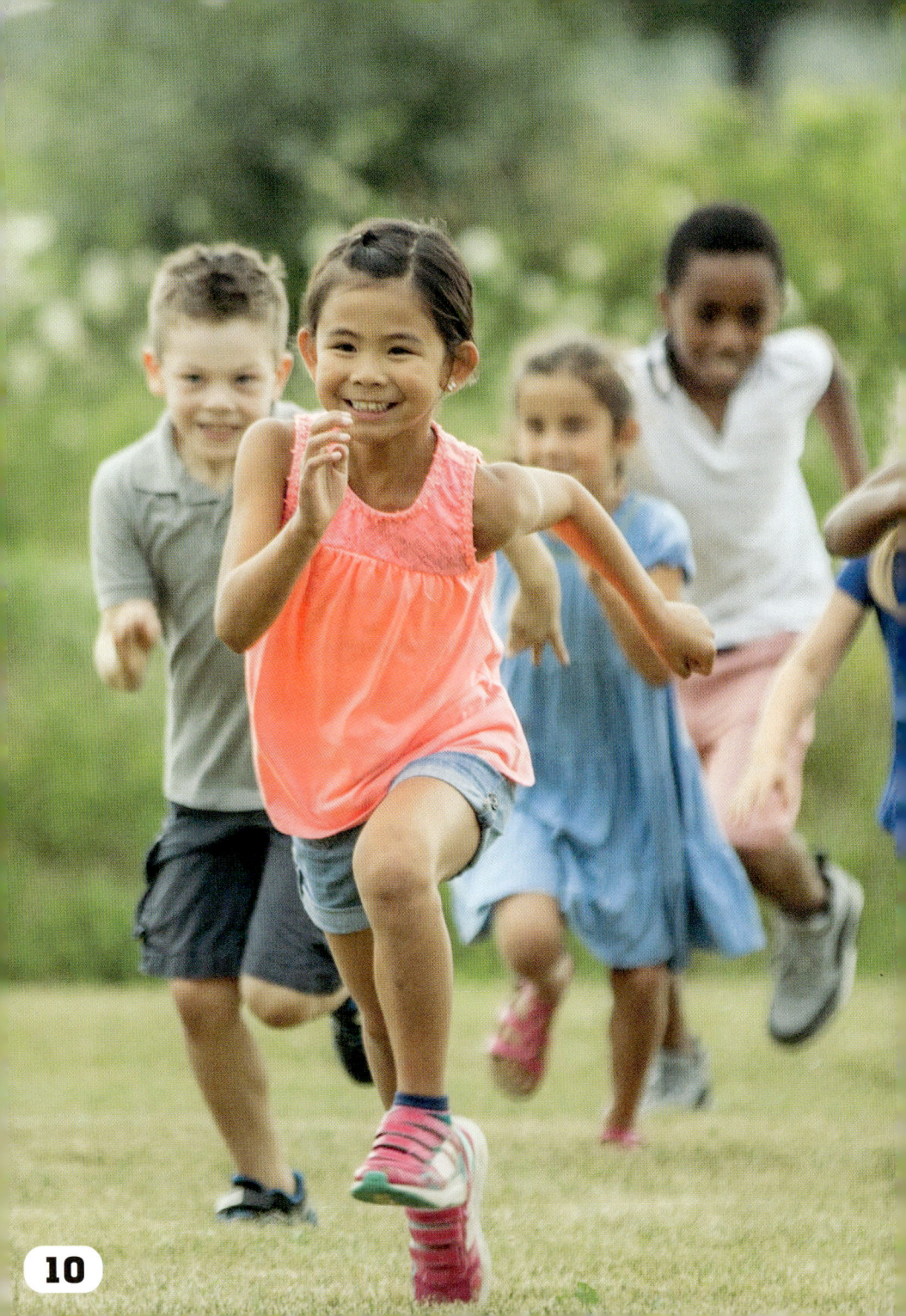

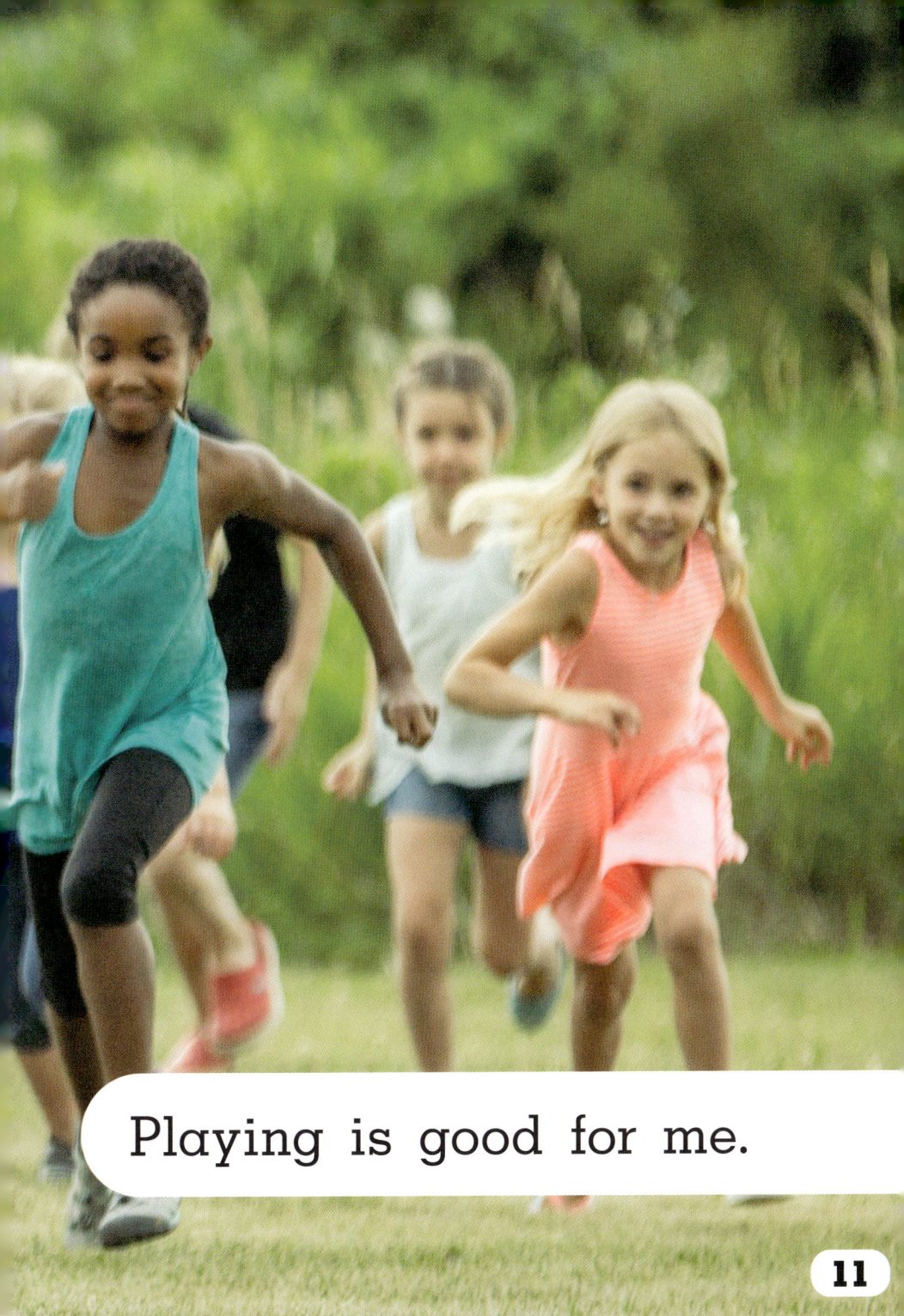

Playing is good for me.

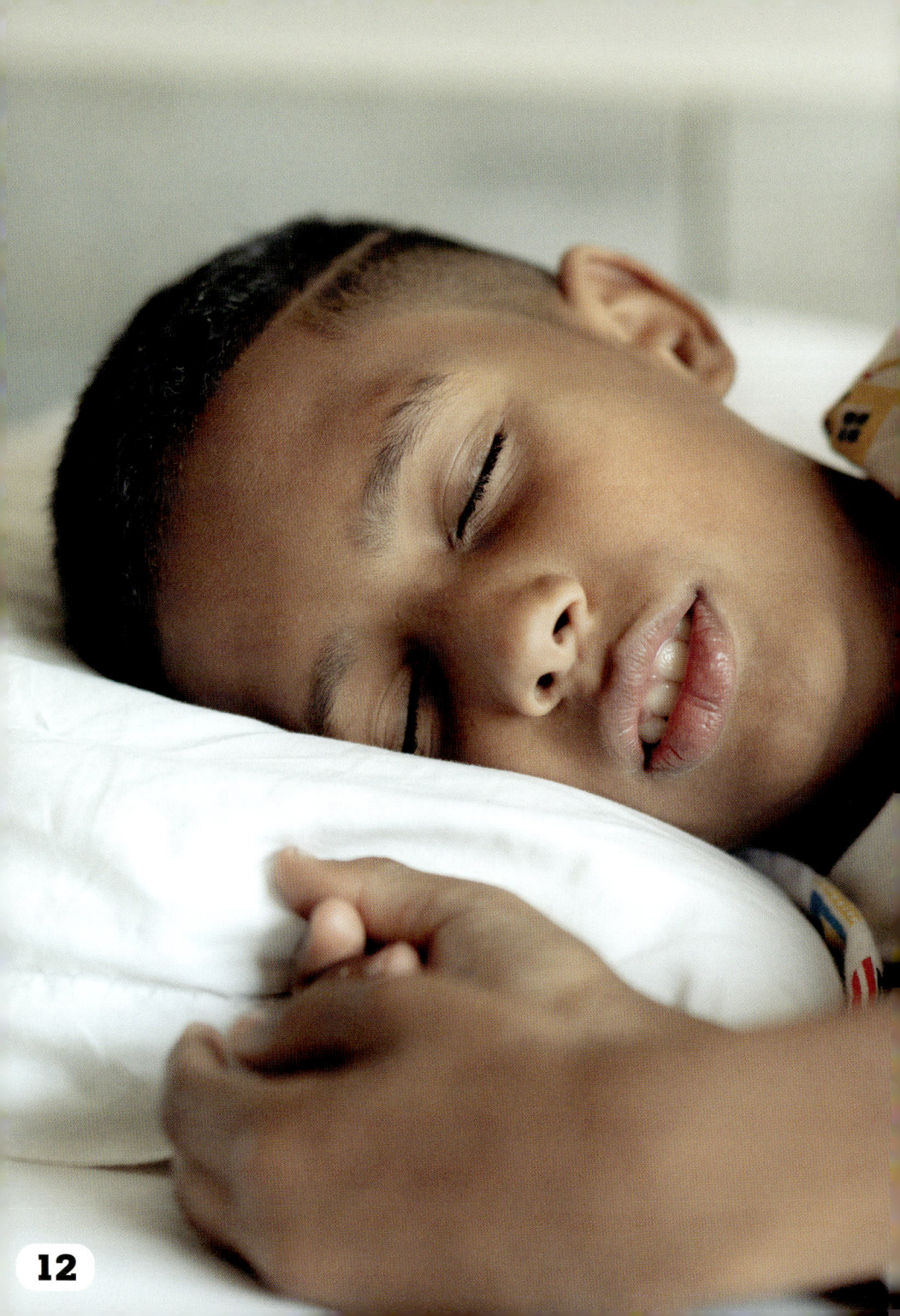

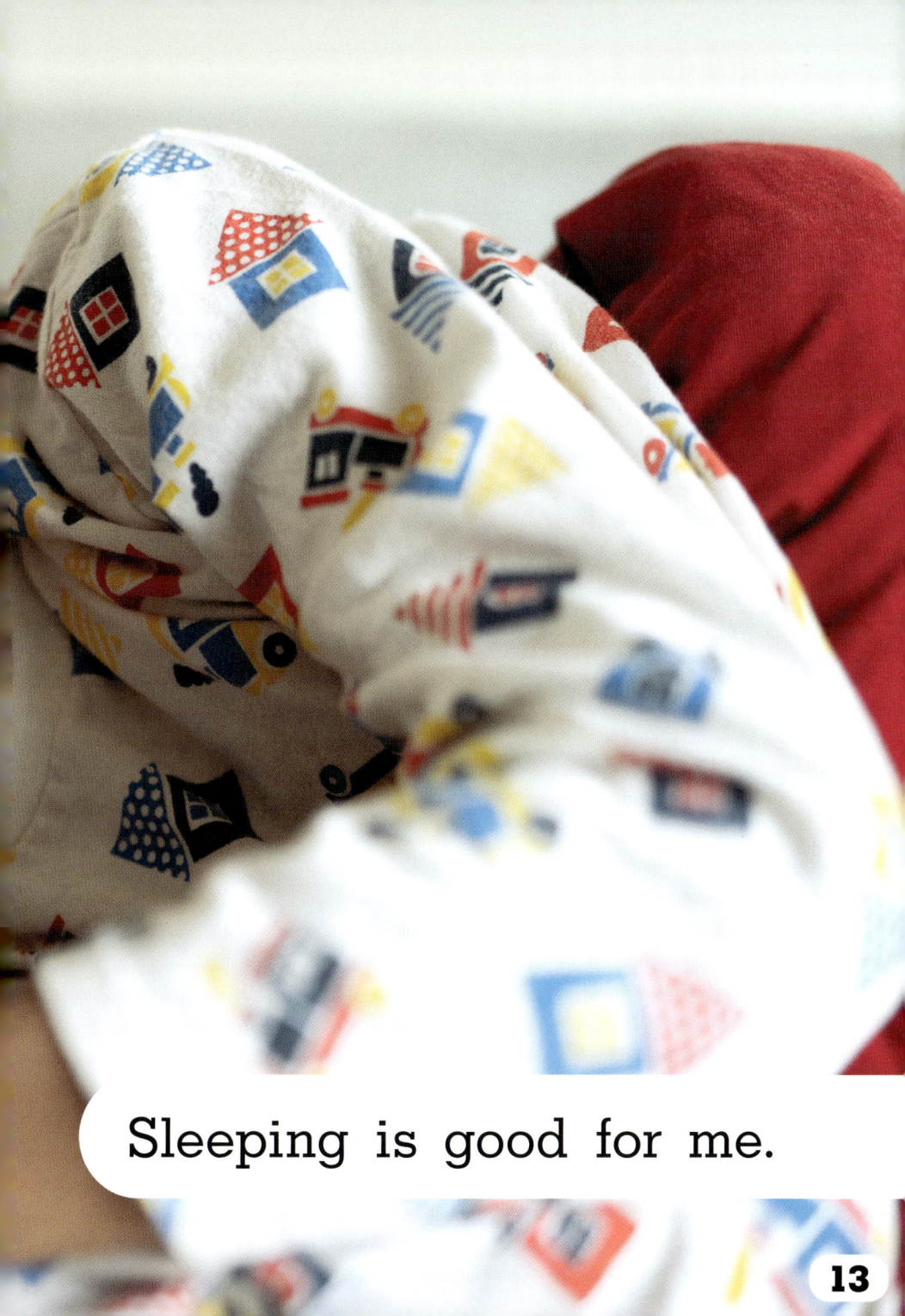

Sleeping is good for me.

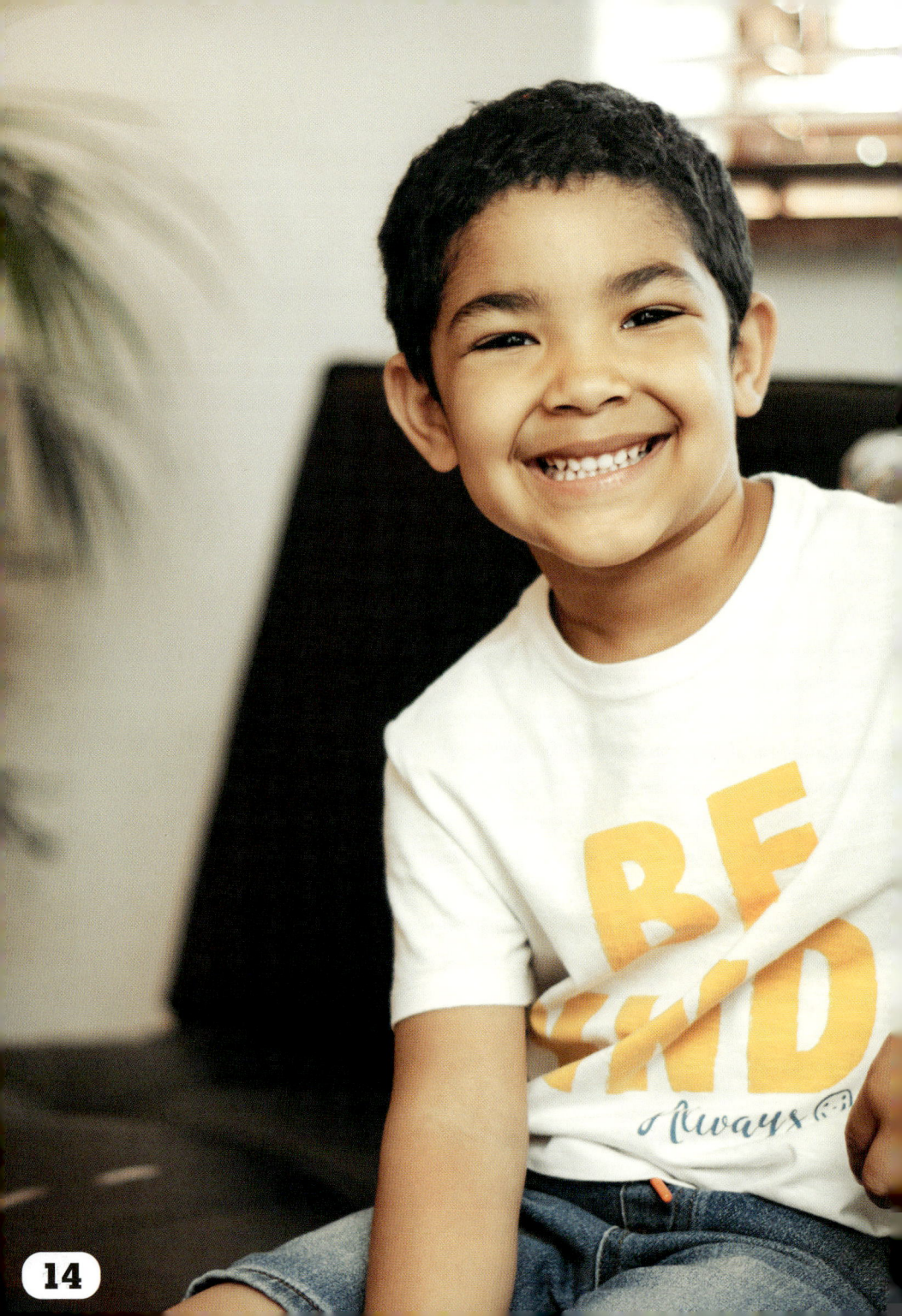

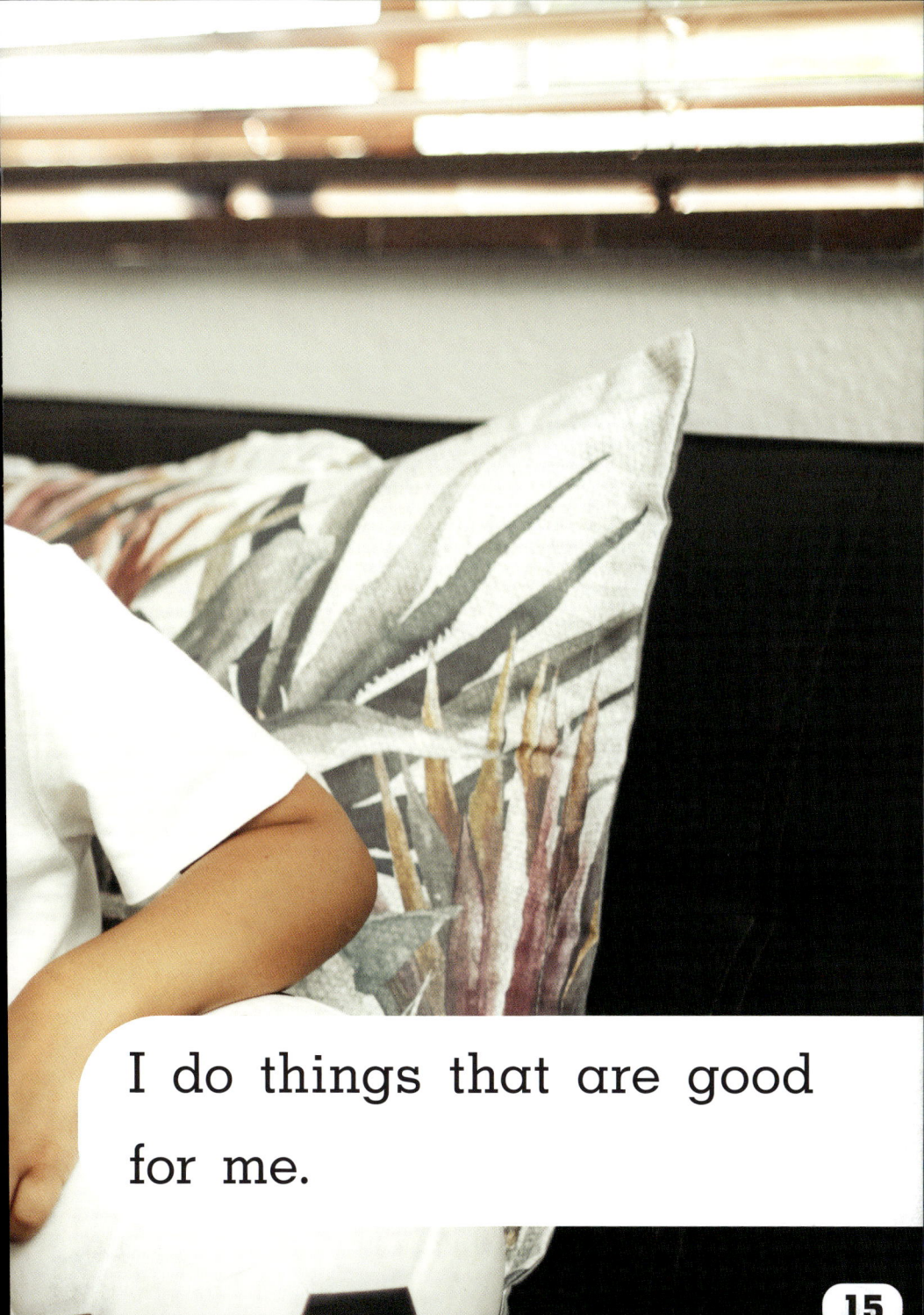

I do things that are good for me.

How do you take care of yourself?

Did You See It?

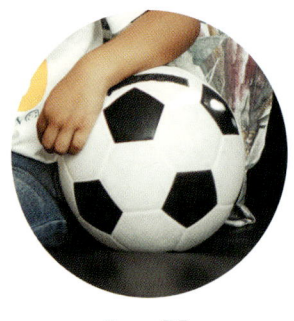
ball

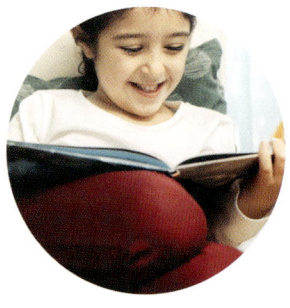
book

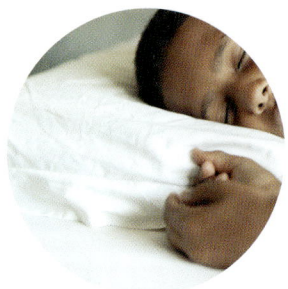
pillow

Index

bathing, 7

dancing, 9

playing, 11

reading, 5

sleeping, 13